Alkaline Diet

— — — — — ❧❦❧ — — — —

The Ultimate Guide to Clean Eating, Weight Loss, and Taking Back Control over Your Health

By Jennifer Sullivan

Table of Contents

Introduction

Few diets out there in the world are perhaps as much effective and misunderstood as the Alkaline Diet! A diet that helps to keep the body healthy by eliminating acid? Surely that sounds pretty absurd, right?

But believe me; once you have completely gone through the book, you are going to look at this diet through a completely different perspective!

Largely known as Alkaline-Ash Diet or even Acid-Ash Diet, the Alkaline Diet basically requires an individual to cut down on certain foods groups that are considered to be extremely "acidic." The goal is to consume a diet that is rich in alkaline produce, such as fruits and vegetables.

While the credibility of the effectiveness of this diet is largely in debate amongst scientists and researchers, the positive impact that thousands of Alkaline Enthusiasts have gained by forming a lifestyle surrounding this diet is just unavoidable!

I am going to let "You" be the judge of this.

As for this book, I have written it in such a way so that it is easily understandable to absolute newcomers who have no idea about the Alkaline Diet, but it also caters for experienced dieters who are looking for something new!

Introduction

The whole book is written in simple, easy to understand language with the information spread across small bite-sized sections perfect for digesting within a few minutes! What's more, I have included more than 30+ recipes for you to experiment and start changing your lifestyle one meal at a time!

I hope that you would find this book helpful and informative. Welcome to the world of the Alkaline Diet!

Chapter 1:

An Overview of the Alkaline Diet

If you have been around and have read all that has been said about the Alkaline Diet, then you have most definitely stumbled upon a number of different pieces of evidence suggesting the extremely positive effects of an alkaline-based diet.

The basic concept of this diet follows the ideology that if acid-forming foods are completely replaced with a diet of only alkaline-based produce, then there will be great improvement in the health conditions of your body. Now, this is obviously a claim, which might seem to be too good to be true! Scientists and experts claim that by following an Alkaline Diet, an individual can easily fend off even the fiercest of diseases such as cancer!

The positive results of an Alkaline Diet have touched the hearts of thousands of people all around the world to the extent where some of them have started to claim that this is nothing short of a miracle!

But we are not simply going to believe in what people speculate, right? If you are planning on going on this diet, then you are going to need some hard evidence to back up your journey, right? That is what we will be looking at in this chapter.

The following chapter will try to explain the complete and overall concept of the Alkaline Diet and help you to judge for yourself if the claims made out there are true or not. However, since this book is also going to be dedicated for beginners and experienced people alike, we are going to start with the very basics of the diet.

Understanding the Philosophy behind the Alkaline Diet

The Alkaline Diet is also synonymously known as Acid-Alkaline or even Alkaline-Ash Diet. The diet is basically based around the concept that the foods which we consume can very easily alter the internal chemistry or acidity and alkalinity of our body by changing the pH of our body. We are going to go into a bit more details here, so bear with me through all the scientific stuff.

Whenever your body starts to metabolize foods and acquire the energy within them, the body is literally burning up the food. The only reason why a literal fire doesn't start up is because the process happens in an extremely slow and gradual fashion. It is strictly controlled by the biological mechanisms of our body.

And where there is fire, there is bound to be ash right? In terms of consumed foods, they also leave behind a residue which we are going to refer to as "Ash."

This "ash" has the potential of either being alkaline, acidic or even neutral. According to researchers, these "ashes" are actually responsible for altering the pH levels of our body. If your body gets high on acidic ash, then your body will immediately start to become more vulnerable and susceptible to various diseases and illnesses.

Alternatively, a high level of alkaline ash is often thought to have a very positive effect on the body which creates a kind of "protective layer" as well. For this reason, it is always strongly recommended that you go for more foods with "alkalizing" properties in them.

The following is a categorization of the different kinds of foods based on the state of their "ashes:"

- **Acidic** - Produce such as meat, fish, poultry, dairy, grains, eggs and even alcohol are considered to be acidic.

- **Neutral** - Foods such as sugars, fats or starches are said to be neutral

- **Alkaline** - Foods including vegetables, legume, nuts and fruits are said to be alkaline.

The Body and pH

The component of our blood which is referred to as "pH" is actually the short form of Potential of Hydrogen. This is essentially a form of measurement to determine if a liquid is either acidic or alkaline. In our case, the liquids are the bodily fluids and tissues.

The measurement is done on a scale of 0 to 14. The lower the value of pH, the more acidic the solution becomes. Consequently, a higher level of pH would indicate a more alkaline solution. The middle point of the scale, pH 7, is considered as a neutral point.

Naturally, our body constitutes of a pH level of 7.4, so from there we are able to deduce that our body stays at its most healthy state whenever the pH level is leaning toward being slightly alkaline. However, it should be noted that the pH level of the body varies throughout the different organs, for example, the stomach is generally regarded as being the most acidic part of our body.

Even if the natural level of pH gets disturbed by a small amount, the body of most organisms, including humans, start to react negatively, which leads to some serious issues. A good example would be the recent increase of carbon dioxide disposition which led to a large a slight decrease in the ocean's pH from 8.2 to 8.1. With this 0.1 change in pH, various aquatic organisms and life forms have started to suffer.

This pH level is not only essential for plant growth, but also the minerals in our food. These minerals are the reason why our body is actually able to maintain its level of pH since the minerals act as buffers. Whenever the level of acidity rises up, minerals start to decrease.

The Impacts of an Un-balanced pH

Now you can clearly see that maintaining a balanced pH in your body is crucial to your well-being and even slight changes can be fatal. If your body starts to become too alkaline, for example, Alkalosis will occur. This is where the body fluids and blood become too alkaline. In this condition, the body will start to experience a sudden loss of electrolytes, lung disease, liver disease, lower oxygen levels, etc.

Chapter 1: An Overview of the Alkaline Diet

Some of the symptoms of Alkalosis include:

- Confusion

- Lightheadedness

- Twitching

- Sudden muscle spasm

- Seizure

- Respiratory problems

- Tingling in facial extremities

Alternatively, if your body starts to get too acidic, then it is said that your body is undergoing "Acidosis". Acidosis has been further divided into several types, which include:

- Metabolic

- Respiratory

- Lactic

- Renal

- Diabetic

Some of the symptoms of Acidosis include:

- Confusion

- Fatigue

- Breathlessness

- Lethargy

Acidosis may very well be induced by a diet containing a lot of animal products with very few fruits and vegetables.

How the Body Protects Itself from pH Changes

Our body is a perfectly designed machine that is capable of taking care of itself to a certain level. This process of self-protection also extends towards protecting itself from sudden changes in the level of pH.

The kidneys of our body are essentially the primary means of defense against acidosis. Whenever the level of acid rises up in our body, the kidneys start to send the excess metabolically-generated acids to our bladder. The waste is then later on excreted when we urinate.

Aside from that, kidneys also help to maintain the levels of bicarbonate, which greatly helps to tackle the acidic effects of the body. However, if for some reason the kidneys start to fail or get compromised, then the body starts to lose control over its pH levels and it becomes more acidic. If this is not taken care of properly at an early stage, the complications will only increase with aging.

However, it should be noted that the filtration process of our kidneys is not the only thing which helps to maintain acid and pH levels. The lungs also play a great role here as well. Carbon dioxide is the by-product of cellular metabolism, but when this CO_2 gets mixed in the bloodstream, blood starts to become acidic. The lungs help out by getting rid of this CO_2 from the body and maintaining a balanced acid-base homeostasis.

With that being said, you must be wondering now how an alkaline diet actually works from a scientific level. Let's take a look at this in the next section!

Research and Working Procedure of the Alkaline Diet

It is important to understand how the Alkaline Diet works, especially for beginners. With that said, here are the key points which you should remember to understand how the Alkaline Diet works, alongside some research data which supports this diet.

- First of all, it is important to note that researchers around the world actually believe that when it comes to the overall acid amount of a regular human diet, there have been significant changes throughout the evolution of humanity. The diet which was followed by the hunters and gatherers was significantly high on chloride, potassium, and magnesium, which are some of the more alkaline electrolytes required by our body to stay healthy. However, thanks to the recent level of industrialization and agricultural advancements, diets these days are much heavier on sodium and low on the essential electrolytes.

- What are the drawbacks of not having those electrolytes? Well, these electrolytes are actually used by our body to maintain the level of pH and tackle acidity whenever we consume something acidic. The kidney plays a great role here in maintaining the electrolyte levels of our body.

- The Journal of Environmental Health Review recently mentioned in one of their articles that the ratio of sodium to potassium in the diets of modern-day people has significantly increased. In fact, the level of potassium in early diets used to vastly outnumber sodium with a score of 10 to 1. However, these days, thanks to the inclusion of "Standard American Diet", people are able to consume potassium and sodium at a ratio of 1:3. This essentially means that people these days are eating 3 times more sodium than potassium!

- There are many adults and children out there today who consume a diet consisting of high sodium, and the saddest part is that the diet which they follow is even lacking other vitamins, minerals, and antioxidants! Furthermore, today's typical Western diet is extremely high in simple sugars, refined fats, chloride, and sodium.

- All of these "evolutionary" changes in the diet of man have resulted in a vast increase of a process known as "metabolic acidosis." This is where, due to the exposure to an uneven form of diet, the pH level of a person fails to maintain at an optimum level. On top of that, today's individuals are also suffering from magnesium and potassium deficiency as well. The deficiency also tends to greatly increase the aging process where organ functions start to deteriorate quickly while bone and tissue mass also starts to waste away. In short, when the body is exposed to a higher level of acid than usual, it slowly starts to drain the body of essential minerals and nutrients. This slowly starts to kill the body from within.

- All of the above symptoms and effects can be avoided by consuming an Alkaline Diet.

With the science of Alkaline Diet out of the way now, it is time make a comparison between one of the most sought after and perhaps well-regarded diet regimen - known as the Paleo Diet - and our very own Alkaline Diet.

Paleo Diet vs. Alkaline Diet

For those of you who are unaware of the Paleo diet, let me give you a quick run-through.

While there are hundreds of different kinds of diet regimens claiming to drastically alter the human physique and help an individual trim down their body fat, very few of them can be said to be effective.

When counting the effective ones, the Ketogenic diet often comes to mind first. But the Paleo diet is slowly climbing up the ladder and has now turned into a total sensation amongst health buffs!

The Paleo diet is a form of diet which dates back to the times of our ancestors, and that is why it is even known as "Caveman Diet", Stone Age Diet or even Primal Diet! This diet tries to answer a very simple question, which is:

"What was the diet of a caveman?"

That answer lies in simply finding out and striking the right balance of calories, carbohydrates, and fats in the diet. Generally speaking, research from the Emory University suggests that it is advisable for people who follow a Paleo diet to take 35% of their total calorie intake from fats, the rest of the 35% from carbohydrates and the final 30% from the proteins.

The Paleo diet basically tries to follow a modern evolutionary version of the diet which was followed by our ancestors. The esteemed author of "The Paleo Diet", Loren Cordain professed that a Paleo diet helps to lessen the amount of glycemic load and results in a healthy ratio of saturated to unsaturated fatty acids. This further enhances the intake of nutrient and vitamins.

With that being said, let us pit Paleo Diet against Alkaline Diet and see how our Alkaline Diet holds up against it.

Both of them aim to water down the risk of malnutrition. Both of them also help to reduce inflammation, aid in digestion and help in losing weight.

Some of the common mechanisms which they share include the elimination of excess sugar, lowering the excess intake of inflammation-inducing omega-6 fatty acids, lowering down or completely eliminating the intake of highly processed carbohydrates or grains, cutting off the consumption of dairy products, and focusing on increasing the consumption of vegetables and fruits.

However, this is where things start to get interesting. When you are going on a Paleo diet, you are forced to cut down on those pesky carbs. You are also denying the body a very good deal of protein, mineral and probiotics sources. Added to that, Paleo diet doesn't necessarily restrict a person to always eating grass-fed or organic foods. Needless to say, the high level of animal protein which the Paleo diet allows isn't a good thing for the body. Beef, cold cuts, chicken, pork, and shellfish can greatly act a source of sulfuric acid in the body since sulfuric acids are produced by breaking down amino acids from proteins.

Alternatively, the Alkaline Diet fully emphasizes on restricting the body to consume only produce that is organically produced. It allows for a degree of probiotics and dairy products such as Kefir or yogurt to be consumed, so the body has no risk of ever being deprived of its essential nutrients. The Alkaline Diet also includes a large quantity of vegetables in its diet. Finally, the Alkaline Diet helps to lower the acidity level of your body.

By now you should have a pretty clear idea of the process and mechanism of the Alkaline Diet. Let us examine in some detail the benefits that you receive when you go on the Alkaline Diet.

Chapter 2:

The Health Benefits of Alkaline Diet

Here are some of the key positive impacts that the Alkaline Diet will have on your body:

1. Helps in protecting the muscle density and bone mass of the body: We have already established the importance of the different types of minerals in our body. They are crucial elements when it comes to maintaining the bone structure of our body as well. In fact, research has shown that eating more vegetables and fruits with alkalizing properties greatly increases the protection against loss of bone and muscle strength due to aging.

The primary route through which the alkaline diet is able to do this is by balancing out the ratio of the essential elements that are required for muscle and bone development. These include magnesium, phosphorous, and calcium. Alkaline Diet also encourages the absorption of Vitamin D and development of growth hormones which further helps to amplify the strength of the bones helps to body to tackle against a number of different persistent diseases.

2. Greatly lowers down the risk of stroke and hypertension: Out of all the effects that an Alkaline Diet has on the body, one of the most potent ones is that it greatly helps to lower down the inflammation caused due to elevation in the levels of growth hormones. The result is improvement of cardiovascular health of the body, wherein the body learns to protect itself from various problems such as high cholesterol build up, kidney stone formation, memory loss, stroke, and hypertension.

3. Greatly minimizes inflammation and chronic pain: Multiple studies have shown that there is a strong connection between a perfectly balanced Alkaline Diet and a decreased level in chronic pain. It has been studied and found that chronic acidosis greatly contributes to problems such as muscle spasms, back pain, menstrual symptoms, headaches, joint pain, and inflammation.

A study performed by a German research institute was able to deduce that whenever patients who were suffering from chronic pain were exposed to a good dosage of Alkaline supplements every day for up to four weeks, they were able to experience extremely satisfying and positive results. In fact, the study confirmed that 76 out of the 82 patients involved experience a marginal decrease in the body's level of pain.

4. Helps to boost the absorption of vitamins and lowers magnesium deficiency: Magnesium is necessary for the proper functioning for at least a hundred different enzymes found in the body. Most people who have suffered from magnesium deficiency have complained that they have experienced significant heart problems, symptoms of insomnia, muscle aches, headaches and also chronic anxiety. Since Alkaline Diet helps to increase the overall magnesium in the body, it helps to mitigate all of these effects. As an added bonus, it also helps to keep away deficiency in vitamin D, which further increases the strength of the immune system and the functioning of the endocrine system.

5. Helps to improve the overall immune functions of the body while protecting it from cancer: When the cells of the body are deprived of minerals required for the proper disposal of waste or providing the body with oxygen, the overall biological architecture of the body starts to suffer. The minerals lost affect the absorption of vitamins, while pathogens and toxins start to gather around the body in this weakened state. Research has shown that the process through which cancerous cells are killed (apoptosis) occurs in a larger percentage in a body which has an overall Alkaline internal environment. On top of that, the shift towards alkalinity is said to be caused by electric charges being altered and release of different components of protein. This action is strongly linked to cancer prevention. Alkalinity in the human body helps to decrease the level of inflammation and lower the risk of disease such as cancer. In addition to that, an alkaline diet is able to offer greater benefits to patients who are undergoing chemotherapy.

6. **Helps in weight loss:** In the Alkaline Diet, you are restricting yourself from the consuming foods that lead to the formation of acid in the body. You are essentially opting for more alkaline-inducing foods. You are actually preparing your body to prevent obesity by lowering the levels of Leptin in your body. This contributes to the reduction of hunger and increase in the fat burning capabilities of our body. In fact, the foods that are suited for the Alkaline Diet are also the very same foods that are high in anti-inflammatory properties! Consuming them helps your body to maintain a normal Leptin level, thus helping the body to feel full after eating just a few calories.

7. Increases the available energy of the body: The pH level of your body affects the cells' ability to produce and process ATP (Adenosine Triphosphate), which is the chemical that supplies your body with energy. If the internal conditions of your body start to get too acidic, then ATP production won't take place properly and soon you will start to feel lethargic from time to time. This can easily be prevented by the consumption of Alkaline Foods to maintain a higher pH.

8. Improves the health of your teeth and gums: If the acid levels around your mouth get too high, it creates an optimum environment for bacteria to grow at a more accelerated rate. These bacteria can result in a number of different complications, including bad breath, gum disease, and tooth decay. Providing a more alkaline condition in your mouth will help the body to decrease the likelihood of these things happening.

9. Slows down the process of aging: Whenever the cells of your body are exposed to a highly acidic environment, they start to lose their proper functionalities. This prevents the cells from repairing themselves properly, which in turn results in accelerated aging. Again, this can be prevented by going on an Alkaline Diet.

10. Enhanced Sexual Drive: After a great deal of research, it has been scientifically proven that acidic conditions in the body lead to decreased sexual performance. This can be avoided by going for foods that are alkaline since an internal alkaline condition will enhance your sexual performance.

Feeling all pumped up yet? Well, we are not done yet. Let us walk through some of the essential tips that will help you easily start pursuing an Alkaline Diet.

Words of Wisdom

If you have made up your mind on following the Alkaline Diet, then there are certain things which you should always remember.

Let's start off with your shopping preference. Whenever you are out in the supermarket buying fresh produce for your next meal, bear in mind to only choose alkaline products that are 100% organic. Experts all around the world believe that this is one the key elements which should always be kept under consideration when pursuing an Alkaline diet.

It is essential to have a good idea of what type of soils were used to grow the vegetables and fruits you are eating. The type of soil greatly influences the alkalinity of the food produced. This information can easily be found by doing a little research on the product which you are buying. However, as a general guide, the best pH for the soil should be around 6 - 7, which allows the plant to absorb optimal levels of the nutrient. If the soil has a pH below 7, then they will be deprived of magnesium and calcium, while a pH above 7 will result in the plant being deprived of manganese, iron, zinc and copper.

Before implementing these tips, though, you might be interested to determine your own pH level! This can be done very easily using a simple pH strip purchased from any pharmaceutical store. Just use the strip with your urine or saliva and compare the color of the strip with the color guide that is provided with the stripe. The most ideal time to check your pH would be the second urine of your morning. As for your saliva, the perfect timing would be to check it one hour prior to consuming a meal or two hours after eating. The ideal pH level of your saliva should range from 8.8 to 7.2

Chapter 3:

The Do's and Don'ts of the Alkaline Diet

While the first chapter had all of the essential information that you are going to need in order to actually dive into the world of Alkaline Diet, this chapter will focus largely on the foods that you are allowed and not allowed to eat. You will also learn some of the more common myths that are associated with the Alkaline Diet.

Let us start off by taking a good look at a list of foods which you are allowed to eat in the Alkaline Diet.

Recommended Foods and Dietary Practices

Fruits and Vegetables

You should always go for fresh vegetables and fruits whenever possible as they tend to promote an increase in the level of alkalinity of your body. Compared to all other food compounds, they are the best source of alkalinity for your blood. There are a number of delicious and interesting one's which you should keep an eye out for. These include:

- Mushroom
- Dates
- Watermelon
- Raisins
- Ripe bananas
- Spinach
- Ginger
- Grapefruit
- Citrus
- Tomatoes
- Avocados
- Summer Black Radish
- Red beet
- Almonds
- Alfalfa Grass
- Celery
- Kale
- Oregano
- Cucumber
- Cabbage
- Jicama
- Endive
- Garlic
- Wheat Grass

- Figs
- Green beans
- Broccoli

Eat Raw Food

It is important to note that you should always try as much as possible to eat your food raw. Now keep in mind here that this is not a recommendation to eat raw meat like a hyena! However, it can't actually be denied that it is always better to go for uncooked vegetables and fruits whenever possible since they are considered as "Biogenic".

When you are cooking your food, you are essentially stripping it off all of the alkalizing minerals. So, try to boost your consumption of raw fruits and vegetables by perhaps juicing them or steaming them lightly for best results.

Go For Plant Proteins

It is ideal that you try to go for some plant proteins as well. Good choices include

- Steamed vegetables

- Almonds

- Lima beans

- Navy beans

Alkaline Water All The Way!

Alkaline waters usually have a pH that ranges from 9 - 11. They can be found in packaged bottles, but as an alternative, you could also go for distilled water as well. It is important that you realize that water filtered through the now much popular "Reverse Osmosis" tends to a bit acidic! So, if you are going for alkalinity, then you are better off with the aforementioned bottled water or tap water. If possible, then you might want to add a few drops of baking soda or lemon to boost the level of alkalinity as well.

Going Green

By now you should be aware that soft drinks and carbonated beverages are strictly forbidden for an alkaline diet. Whenever you feel that you truly crave a sip of soda, then you are better off going for drinks that are derived from grasses or green vegetables.

If possible, then you can also look for them in powdered form, as they are filled with f alkaline-inducing chlorophyll. Keep in mind that chlorophyll has a very similar structure to that of human blood and therefore greatly enhances the alkalinity of the blood as well.

Good enough so far?

Now if you are really dedicated, then you should most definitely try to avoid the following foods and habits. They will simply increase the level of acidity in your body.

Foods and Dietary Habits to Avoid

As always, it is important to first focus on those foods that you absolutely must stay away from. So, in general, you should try to avoid:

- Processed foods that are high in sodium. These kinds of foods tend to cause the blood vessels to become constricted.

- Conventional meats or cold cut meats

- Lentils

- Eggs

- Processed cereals such as Corn Flakes

- Alcohol and caffeinated beverages

- Rice, pasta or any other packaged grain products. When we talk of grains, we are referring to all kinds of grains, regardless of whether they are whole grain or not.

- Products that are extremely rich in calcium can lead to severe cases of Osteoporosis! And this is because they are potent in creating an extremely acidic condition inside the body. If your blood stream starts to become more acidic, your body begins to dissolve the calcium from the bones in order to create a balance with the pH level. Leafy vegetables are therefore the way to go when it comes to tackling osteoporosis.

- Walnuts and Peanuts

Aside from the foods listed above, there are also some habits which you should try to avoid. These include:

- Use of drugs or alcohol

- Consumption of large quantities of caffeine

- Use of a large number of antibiotics

- Consumption of artificial sweeteners

- Not exercising

- Going for excess animal meat mostly from inorganic sources

- Ingestion of hormones through artificial means such as medicines or beauty products

- Exposing your body to radiation from cleaners, computers, microwaves, cell phones

- Chronic stress

- Using preservatives of any form of food coloring

- Getting exposed to herbicides or pesticides

- Extreme cases of pollution

- Eating refined or processed foods

- Breathing shallowly

De-Bunking the Acid-Ash Myth of Osteoporosis

First off, keep in mind that osteoporosis is a bone disease that is classified as the process through which bones start to lose their mineral content. This is particularly common amongst women who are undergoing menopause, and it increases the risk of fractures in elderly women.

Chapter 3: The Do's and Don'ts of the Alkaline Diet

Many individuals who pursue the Alkaline Diet believe that if you want to maintain a constant pH of blood, then the body takes away essential alkaline minerals from the bones to effectively negate the side effects of acid. So basically, what they claim is that the acid in our body is being tackled by sacrificing the minerals of our bone.

Following this theory, it is also claimed that a diet that leads to the formation of acidic conditions in the body, including the standard Western one, will simply lead to a loss of bone density and minerals. This is also known as the "Acid-Ash Hypothesis of Osteoporosis"

But what most people fail to realize, is that there is a huge gaping hole in this theory which completely ignores the role of the kidney in this process! Sacrificial bones aside, our kidneys are the most fundamental and core organs that are responsible for the removal of acids from our body in order to regulate the pH.

Whenever the levels of acids tend to rise up, our kidney starts to produce bicarbonate ions, which help to neutralize the acids and regulate the pH of our blood. At the same time, the respiratory system is also working closely in order to remove the carbon dioxide from the blood stream as well.

But that's not all! There's another problem with this theory. It completely ignores the core driver of osteoporosis, which is the loss of a bone protein known as "Collagen". The loss of collagen is actually linked to low levels of ascorbic and orthosilicic acid.

Research done by Zero Observational Studies found that there is a strong link between dietary acid and the bone density of our body, but there is no relation at all between the pH and the health of our bone. This contradicts the popular belief! Acid forming diets are actually helpful to bone formation and do not lead to its destruction.

The reason why this has been brought that up is because you should always understand that not all claims made by people out there are true. You should always keep yourself abreast of any hoaxes.

The above debunking of the acid-ash hypothesis is not an endorsement of an acidic diet! The aim here is to show you that sometimes a balance between the two might be needed to be struck in order to maintain optimal results, depending on your physique and health conditions.

Chapter 4:

Breakfast Recipes

The Classical Breakfast Quinoa

Serving: 4

Prep Time: 5 minutes

Cooking Time: 15 minutes

Ingredients:

- 1 cup of quinoa

- 2 cups of water

- 2-inch cinnamon sticks

- 3 tablespoons of maple syrup

For added flavor:

- ½ cup of blueberries, raspberries or strawberries

- 2 tablespoon of raisins

- 1 teaspoon of lime

- ¼ teaspoon of freshly grated nutmeg

- 3 tablespoons of whipped coconut cream

- 2 tablespoons of chopped cashew nuts

- Yoghurt if desired

Instructions:

Take a fine strainer and pass the grain through it. Strain them very well and then proceed to rinse them with water.

Take a medium-sized saucepan and pour in the water alongside the strained grains and bring the mixture to a boil.

Toss in the cinnamon sticks then and cover it up.

Lower the heat and let it simmer for about 15 minutes or until liquid is nicely absorbed.

Remove the heat and fluff the mixture up using a fork.

Toss in the cinnamon alongside the maple syrup for added flavor.

If you want more flavor, then add in any of the above ingredients listed under "For added flavor."

Nutrition Values

Calories: 223

Fats: 5 g

Carbs: 37 g

Fiber: 8 g

Roughly Cut Oats of Steel

Serving: 4

Prep Time: 5 minutes

Cooking Time: 15 minutes

Ingredients:

- 3 ¾ cups water
- 1 ¼ cup of steel-cut oats
- ¼ teaspoon salt

For added flavor:

- 1 teaspoon of cinnamon
- ½ teaspoon of nutmeg
- ½ teaspoon of lemon pepper
- 1 teaspoon of Garam masala
- Mixed berries
- Diced mangos
- Sliced bananas
- Dried Fruits
- Nuts

For creaminess:

- 1 tablespoon of coconut milk

Instructions:

Take a medium sized saucepan and pour in the water and put it over high heat.

Stir in the steel-cut oats then alongside the specified amount of salt.

Gently lower the heat to a medium-low setting and let it simmer for at least 25 minutes until nicely thickened.

Make sure to keep stirring it from time to time.

Toss in the coconut milk or almond butter for an added flavor. (You can also choose from the above options for your flavor).

Once done, serve with some delicious berries or nuts of your choosing.

Nutrition Values

Calories: 231

Fats: 5g

Carbs: 38g

Fiber: 6g

Tantalizing Sunchoke Hash

Serving: 4

Prep Time: 10 minutes

Cooking Time: 6 minutes

Ingredients:

- 4 pieces of finely sliced and well-blanched Sunchokes
- 6 Brussels sprouts, thinly sliced
- Seas salt as needed
- Ground pepper as needed
- Drizzle of truffle oil or extra virgin olive oil with Rosemary infused in
- Finely sliced spring onion for garnish

Instructions:

Take a bowl and fill it up with cold water.

Plunk in your Sunchokes into the bowl of cold water right after slicing them up.

Rinse them thoroughly with the water three times and then pat them very gently. This will help the Sunchokes to slow down the oxidation process and keep them colorless.

Take a pan and put it over medium heat and pour in some ghee or oil.

Toss in the sliced up Brussels sprouts alongside the Sunchokes and sauté them for 4 minutes finely until both of them are finely cooked up.

Once done, take them out and serve.

Nutrition Values

Calories: 279

Fats: 18 g

Carbs: 28 g

Fiber: 3 g

The Perfect Cucumber Salad from China

Serving: 4

Prep Time: 15 minutes

Cooking Time: 0 minutes

Ingredients:

- 1 lbs of fresh cucumber

- 4 cloves of garlic

- 3 tablespoon of sesame seed oil

- Pinch of salt

- Pinch of pepper

Instructions

Take a bowl and pour in the oil. Mix in a pinch of pepper and salt.

Toss in the minced garlic and add to the bowl. Mix it with the other ingredients.

Wash up your cucumbers then and cut them up into halves and cut the halves into thin slices.

Toss in the slices in your mix.

Chill them in your fridge for about 10 minutes.

Serve chilled.

Nutrition Values

Calories: 20

Fats: 0 g

Carbs: 4 g

Fiber: 1 g

A Fine Quinoa Pasta Dish With Lovely Artichoke Sauce

Serving: 4

Prep Time: 15 minutes

Cooking Time: 20 minutes

Ingredients:

- 7 oz. pasta
- 8 oz. frozen artichoke
- 5 oz. fresh tomatoes
- 1 medium sized onion
- 1 clove of garlic
- 1 oz. pine nuts
- 1 teaspoon of yeast free vegetable stock
- 3 tablespoon of fresh basil
- ½ teaspoon of yeast free vegetable stock
- 3 tablespoons of fresh basil
- ½ teaspoon of organic sea salt
- 1 pinch of cayenne pepper
- 2 tablespoons of cold pressed extra virgin olive oil

Instructions

Start off by preparing your artichokes and cooking them until tender. Cook the pasta by following the instructions on the packet.

In the meantime, chop up all the tomatoes into cubes and chop up the onions, basil and garlic into small sized pieces.

Heat up about 2 tablespoons of olive oil and pour them into a pan.

Toss in the pine nuts and stir-fry them alongside the garlic, onion for a few minutes.

In about ½ a cup of water dissolve your yeast free vegetable stock and then add that to the pan as well.

Simmer for about 2 minutes and keep stirring it from time to time.

Finally, add in the basil and season it with some salt and cayenne pepper.

Pour the finely created sauce over your pasta and serve hot.

Nutrition Values

Calories: 286

Fats: 13 g

Carbs: 26 g

Fiber: 3 g

Chapter 5:

Lunch Recipes

Great Indian Lentil Curry

Serving: 4-6

Prep Time: 10 minutes

Cooking Time: 10 minutes

Ingredients:

- 1 cup fine red lentils
- 2 green chilies
- ½ teaspoon of cumin seeds
- ½ teaspoon of turmeric
- 1-inch piece of grated ginger
- 1 clove of garlic, minced
- 1 medium onion, sliced
- 2 medium tomatoes
- 1 tablespoon of oil

- Salt as needed

- Chopped up cilantro for garnish

- Lime juice as preferred

Instructions:

Start off by taking a bowl and filling it up with water. Toss in your lentils and soak them for at least 6 hours.

Take a pan and place it over a low flame. Pour in the water and the lentils and boil them with a pinch of turmeric. Make sure to keep the texture thick enough for your satisfaction.

Simmer off the excess moisture. Once done, take out and place them in a bowl. Using a potato masher, mash them all up nicely and keep on one side.

Take another pan and heat up your oil. Toss in the onions followed by garlic, cumin, ginger and the remaining turmeric.

Toss in the tomatoes, chilies alongside some salt and cook them finely until nicely done. Toss in the previously prepared lentils then and bring the whole mixture to a nice boil. Once it has reached boiling state, take it off the stove and squeeze in some lime juice

Garnish the dish with touches of cilantro and serve with some rice

Nutrition Values

Calories: 421

Fats: 6 g

Chapter 5: Lunch Recipes

Carbs: 79 g

Fiber: 59 g

A Slightly Spicy Savory of Vegetables

Serving: 4-6

Prep Time: 10 minutes

Cooking Time: 10 minutes

Ingredients:

- 2 tablespoons of vegetable oil

- 1 chopped up large sized onion

- 1 Poblano chili, seeded and chopped

- 1 red bell pepper, seeded and chopped

- 3 cloves of garlic, minced

- 1 ½ teaspoons of chili powder

- 1 ½ teaspoons of cumin powder

- 2 cups of cooked bean, rinsed and drained

- 2 ½ cups vegetable stock

- 3 teaspoon of lime juice

- 4 tablespoon of chopped up cilantro

Instructions:

Take a cooking pot and place over medium heat. Pour in your oil to heat it up and then toss in the onions only to sauté them nicely.

Once done, toss in the red bell pepper garlic, jalapeno and Poblano chili. Let it cook for about 2-3 minutes until all of the vegetables are finely tender.

Next, add in the spices and stir them all up gently. Add in the beans alongside the vegetable stock.

Bring the whole mixture to a boil and cook it over medium-high temperature for approximately 15 minutes. Stir in the lemon juice then and sprinkle some cilantro as garnish

Pro Tip: If you want to make the dish more delicious, then you can some additional ingredients such as cabbage, mushroom, burdock, sweet potatoes etc. right before tossing in the beans. Just make sure not to add any kind of dairy, sugar or meat products as they might hamper the alkalinity of the recipe.

Nutrition Values:

Calories: 485

Fats: 13 g

Carbs: 71 g

Fiber: 12 g

Assorted Wild Garlic – Avocado Salad

Serving: 2

Prep Time: 10 minutes

Cooking Time: 0 minutes

Ingredients:

- 1 avocado, peeled

- 1 bunch of wild garlic

- 3 tomatoes

- 1 red bell pepper

- 2 tablespoon of cold pressed extra virgin olive oil

- Sea salt as needed

- Pinch of cayenne pepper

Instructions:

Cut up your peeled avocado and toss them into a bowl. Chop up the bell pepper into halves and then further into thin slices.

Chop up your tomatoes into small cubes and place them in a medium-sized bowl. Chop up your wild garlic into very fine pieces and place them in the bowl.

Pour in some olive oil in that mix and mix it well. Toss in some pepper and salt to make sure that the flavor is fine.

Enjoy your salad!

Nutrition Values:

Calories: 213

Fats: 21 g

Carbs: 2 g

Fiber: 5 g

A Beautiful Zucchini Salad

Serving: 2

Prep Time: 10 minutes

Cooking Time: 0 minutes

Ingredients

- 1 fresh Zucchini
- 1 red bell pepper
- 2 tomatoes
- 1 onion
- 1 clove of garlic
- ½ a fresh lemon
- 2 tablespoons of cold pressed extra virgin olive oil
- Pinch of salt
- Pinch of pepper
- 1 teaspoon of fresh herbs

Instructions

Wash up your Zucchini first and cut up the upper portion and the bottom part. Cut them up in lengthwise halves and slice them up crosswise.

Wash up and dice your tomatoes. Then wash the bell pepper and cut them in half, followed by cutting in slices.

Chapter 5: Lunch Recipes

Cut up your onions then and turn them into rings.

Toss in your vegetables in a medium sized salad bowl.

Take another small sized bowl and mix in the lemon juice, olive oil, minced up garlic, fresh herbs alongside some pepper and salad as needed.

Pour the mixture over your salad and mix gently.

Enjoy this beautiful salad!

Nutrition Values

Calories: 35

Fats: 7 g

Carbs: 7 g

Fiber: 1 g

Stir Fried Tofu Vegetables and Coconut Milk

Serving: 4

Prep Time: 10 minutes

Cooking Time: 5 minutes

Ingredients

- 1 lbs tofu

- 3 medium-sized Zucchinis

- 3 tomatoes

- 1 red bell pepper

- 1 green bell pepper

- ½ lbs green beans

- 1 ½ cups of fresh coconut milk

- 2 tablespoons of cold pressed extra virgin olive oil

- Sea salt as needed

- Pepper as needed

- ½ a tablespoon of curry powder

- ¼ tablespoon of ginger

- Fresh assorted selection of Herbs

Instructions

Dice up your tofu and chop the Zucchinis.

Chop your pepper bells, beans and tomatoes into bite-sized portions.

Take a pan and pour in some oil.

Toss in your tofu to fry them up for a few minutes. Toss in the bell pepper, zucchini, and beans. Then stir-fry them for a few minutes

Toss in the tomatoes then alongside the coconut milk and stir them well yet again and let it cook for a few minutes more.

Finally, season it with some pepper, salt, ginger, curry powder and your favorite herbs if possible.

Serve the mixture with some wild rice of soba noodles.

Enjoy!

Nutrition Values

Calories: 210

Fats: 17 g

Carbs: 8 g

Fiber: 3 g

Multi-Cultured Pumpkin Potato Patties

Serving: 2

Prep Time: 10 minutes

Cooking Time: 5 minutes

Ingredients

- 1 lbs pumpkin

- 1 lb potatoes

- 2.5 oz. soy flour

- 4 tablespoons of water

- 3 tablespoon of chopped up parsley

- Sea salt as needed

- Organic salt as needed

- Pinch of pepper

- Cold pressed extra virgin olive oil

Instructions

Peel off the skin of your pumpkin and potatoes.

Take a grater and grate them up into nice chunky pieces.

Mix in about 2 tablespoons of soy flour with 4 tablespoons of water in a bowl.

Put in your grated potatoes alongside the pumpkin with the rest of the soy flour in another bowl.

Add in the flour water mixture to it then and mix everything finely.

Season it with some pepper, salt and parsley.

Take a pan and heat up some oil.

Using the previously made mixture, form a number of patties and fry them up for 2-3 minutes.

Serve hot.

Nutrition Values

Calories: 375

Fats: 16 g

Carbs: 46 g

Fiber: 7 g

Fine Leek Fry from Italy

Serving: 2

Prep Time: 10minutes

Cooking Time: 20 minutes

Ingredients

- 2 silvered stalks of leeks

- 2 diced up middle sized white onion

- 1 silvered Zucchini

- 2 coarsely diced up tomatoes

- 2 tablespoon of extra virgin olive oil

- 1 tablespoon of grated cheddar

- 1 teaspoon of sea salt

- 1 tablespoon of parsley

- 1 teaspoon of oregano

- ½ a teaspoon of curry powder

- Freshly ground black pepper

- ½ a cup of water

Instructions

Take a medium sized pan and heat up some oil in it. Toss in your onions and saute to lightly brown them.

Toss in the Zucchinis and cook them for around 3-4 minutes. Pour in the water and cover it with a lid. Reduce the heat to low and simmer for about 10 minutes.

Toss in your tomatoes then and season with some curry and pepper.

Cook for yet another 10 minutes, making sure that the pan is covered up. Once the food is ready, season it up with some extra salt and parsley.

Toss in some cheese as well if you want just before serving it.

If possible, serve with some alkaline bread for added effect.

Nutrition Values

Calories: 80

Fats: 7 g

Carbs: 4 g

Fiber: 1 g

Celery Mixed Almond Salad

Serving: 2

Prep Time: 60 minutes

Cooking Time: 0 minutes

Ingredients

- 10 oz. sliced celery

- 7 oz. apples, cubed

- 2/3 cups water

- 1/3 cup almonds

- ½ a lemon

- ½ tablespoon of salt

- Pepper as needed

Instructions

Take a medium sized bowl and toss in the apples, celery with some lemon juice and mix them well. Blend up all of the almonds and mix them up with water until you have a very smooth paste.

Place the paste in a bowl and season with some pepper and salt. Mix them well and let it refrigerate for an hour.

Mix the past with the previously cut apples and celery and serve chilled.

Nutrition Values

Calories: 221

Fats: 15 g

Carbs: 23 g

Fiber: 3 g

Chapter 6:

Dinner Recipes

Greatly Wild Rice with Alkalizing Vegetables

Serving: 4

Prep Time: 10 minutes

Cooking Time: 5 minutes

Ingredients

- 1 cup of wild rice
- 1 cup of Pak Choi
- 1 cup of Broccoli
- 1 cup of Young Beans
- 2 cups carrots
- 1 cup of bean sprout
- ½ cup of vegetable broth
- 1 chili
- 1 fresh juice of lime

- Cilantro as needed

- Basil as required

- Seas Salt as required

Instructions

Start off this recipe by chopping up the Pak Choi, beans, carrots, broccoli and bean sprouts. Then toss them in a pan.

Pour in some vegetable broth and steam fry them until finely cooked but still a bit crunchy.

In the meantime, pound the cilantro alongside the finely chopped up chili. Pour in the lime juice then to create your perfect dressing.

Put some rice on a platter and toss in the prepared green vegetables. Cover them up with your dressing and serve hot!

Nutrition Values

Calories: 200

Fats: 2 g

Carbs: 33 g

Fiber: 2 g

Assorted Dish Of Stir Fried Tofu and Soba Noodles

Serving: 4

Prep Time: 10 minutes

Cooking Time: 5 minutes

Ingredients

- 16 oz. Buckwheat Soba Noodles

- 1 packet of firm tofu

- 1 green or red pepper bell

- 1 small cup of bean sprouts

- 1 small cup of Pak Choi

- 1 onion

- 1 garlic clove

- Yeast-free vegetable broth

- Sea salt as needed

- Pepper as needed

- Ginger as needed

Instructions

Open the pack of your noodles and cook according to the directions specified on the packaging.

Once you are done with the noodles, cut up your tofu into tiny bite-sized pieces and toss them in a pan with some vegetable broth.

Saute them for a few minutes and place them on the side for later use. Toss in your chopped up pepper, onion, Pak Choi, garlic, bean sprouts and stir fry them for about 5 minutes in your pan.

Add some vegetable broth if you wish. Toss in the noodles in that mixture then alongside the previously prepared tofu.

Sprinkle pinches of pepper, salt and ginger and mix them well.

Serve hot.

Nutrition Values

Calories: 683

Fats: 41 g

Carbs: 63 g

Fiber: 4 g

A Spicy Tofu Burger

Serving: 4

Prep Time: 5 minutes

Cooking Time: 15 minutes

Ingredients

- 16 oz. tofu

- 4 oz. green bell peppers, chopped

- 6 teaspoon of organic chili sauce

- ½ teaspoon of sea salt

- 2 teaspoon of extra virgin olive oil

- Pepper as needed

Instructions

Chop up your tofu first alongside the bell pepper, onions into tiny pieces.

Take a pan and pour in some oil and toss in the previously cut onions and bell pepper to stir fry them nicely for 5 minutes. Toss in the tofu then and stir fry them together for another 15 minutes.

Add the chili sauce to the mix alongside some pepper and salt according to your taste. Add in some water just to make the mixture a little bit wet. Use alkaline bread and spread the mixture in between to form your burger

Nutrition Values

Calories: 496

Fats: 13 g

Carbs: 74 g

Fiber: 6 g

Healthy Pasta with a Special Tomato and Pepper Sauce

Serving: 4

Prep Time: 5 minutes

Cooking Time: 10 minutes

Ingredients

- 16 oz. vegetable pasta

- 10 oz. tomatoes

- ½ cup of sun dried tomatoes

- 1 small red bell pepper

- 1 small Zucchini

- 1 onion

- 2 garlic cloves

- 1 chili

- 5 fresh basil leaves

- 3 tablespoon of cold pressed olive oil

- Sea salt as needed

- Pepper as needed

Instructions

Start off by cooking your vegetable pasta according to the instructions given on the packaging.

Cut up the tomatoes, zucchini, and bell pepper into fine cubes and then chop up the onions, chili and garlic.

Take a pan and pour in some oil to heat it up. Toss in the onion, chili, garlic and pepper and fry it for a few minutes.

Toss in the tomatoes, zucchini then and let them cook for another 5-10 minutes.

Finally, add in some basil alongside salt and pepper for added flavor.

Gently place your pasta on top of a plate and garnish it with some sauce and another seasoning if you wish.

Serve hot.

Nutrition Values

Calories: 591

Fats: 22 g

Carbs: 73 g

Fiber: 5 g

A Superb Alkaline Salad from The Mediterranean

Serving: 3

Prep Time: 10 minutes

Cooking Time: 0 minutes

Ingredients

- 1 piece of red bell pepper
- 1 piece of yellow bell pepper
- 3 large tomatoes
- 10 black olives, dipped in oil
- 1 onion
- 1 small leek
- Celery leaves

For Dressing

- 1/3 cup of fresh lemon juice
- ¾ cup of cold pressed olive oil
- 1 teaspoon of garlic powder
- ½ teaspoon of ground oregano
- ¼ teaspoon of dried rosemary
- 1 teaspoon of dried basil
- ½ teaspoon of ground cumin

- A dash of sea salt

- A dash of cayenne pepper

Instructions

Dice up your tomatoes and pepper. Cut up the onion, celery leaves and leeks into fine strips.

Take a salad bowl and toss in the prepared vegetables. For the salad dressing, toss in the all of the listed ingredients under "For Dressing" in a blender and let them mix up until they are finely emulsified.

Season them with some flaxseed if you thicker dressing. Toss in the dressing over your vegetables and mix them up.

Serve.

Nutrition Values

Calories: 204

Fats: 16 g

Carbs: 10 g

Fiber: 1 g

Emmenthal Soup with Cauliflowers from Switzerland

Serving: 2

Prep Time: 5 minutes

Cooking Time: 5 minutes

Ingredients

- 2 cups of cauliflower pieces

- 1 cubed up potato

- 2 cups of yeast free vegetable stock

- 3 tablespoon of cubed up Emmenthal cheese

- 2 tablespoon of fresh chives

- 1 tablespoon of pumpkin seeds

- 1 pinch of nutmeg

- 1 pinch of cayenne pepper

Instructions

Cook up your cauliflower and the potatoes in the vegetable stock until they are tender. Take them out and toss them in a blender and blend until fully pureed.

Season your soup with some nutmeg, cayenne and a bit pepper and salt if you like.

Toss in the Emmenthal cheese alongside the chives and stir them for a few minutes until the total mixture is completely smooth and ready.

Garnish it up with some pumpkin seeds.

Serve hot.

Nutrition Values

Calories: 351

Fats: 14 g

Carbs: 28 g

Fiber: 4 g

Buckwheat Pasta mixed up with Bell Pepper and Broccoli

Serving: 3-4

Prep Time: 5 minutes

Cooking Time: 10 minutes

Ingredients

1. 16 oz. Buckwheat pasta
2. 4 tablespoons of extra virgin olive oil cold pressed out
3. 2 cloves of garlic, diced
4. 1 middle-sized white onion ring
5. 1 red bell pepper
6. 1 broccoli head, cut up into florets
7. 3 medium tomatoes, sliced
8. 3 carrots, sliced
9. 1 tablespoon of fresh lemon juice
10. 1 teaspoon of oregano
11. 1 teaspoon of yeast-free vegetable broth
12. Sea salt as needed
13. Pepper as needed

Instructions

Start off by cutting up all of your vegetables and preparing them for cooking.

Take a pot of water and heat up your salt water and cook your Buckwheat pasta alongside the broccoli in another pot.

In the meantime, heat up about 2 tablespoons of olive oil over medium heat in a pan. Toss in the onions and garlic and sauté them nicely until a translucent texture is seen.

Take out this mix and keep them in a pan aside. Place about 2 tablespoons of olive oil on the same pan and cook your vegetables until they are finely tender.

Cook them in this order – carrots followed by bell pepper and then tomatoes. Once done, toss in the drained up broccoli and the onions to that pan and season them with some lemon juice, vegetable broth, oregano and pepper/salt.

Stir them finely and taste well. Mix in this vegetable mixture over you alkaline buckwheat pasta and serve hot.

Nutrition Values

Calories: 583

Fats: 26 g

Carbs: 61 g

Fiber: 4 g

Classical Ratatouille For Alkaline Diet

Serving: 4

Prep Time: 5 minutes

Cooking Time: 8 minutes

Ingredients

- 5 tomatoes

- 1 large Zucchini

- 1 large eggplant

- 1 green bell pepper

- 1 large onion

- 2 garlic cloves

- 2 teaspoons of herbs de Provence

- 3 tablespoons of cold pressed extra virgin olive oil

- Pinch of sea salt

- Pinch of pepper

- 1 cup of alkaline water

Instructions

Start off by scrubbing off your vegetables and washing them up nicely. Dice up the pepper bell, tomatoes and slice up your Zucchinis alongside the eggplants.

Then slice up the garlic and onion into thin slices. Take a pot and pour in some olive oil. Heat the olive oil over medium heat. Toss in the garlic, onions and saute them a few minutes.

Add in the eggplants and Zucchini slices them alongside the pepper bell and stir fry the whole mix for about 8 minutes.

Pour in the cup of water and mix up the tomatoes, herb and stir them finely for an extra 2 or 3 minutes until the vegetables are all tender.

Taste it and add some extra salt or pepper if you want.

Serve hot.

Nutrition Values

Calories: 160

Fats: 10 g

Carbs: 19 g

Fiber: 5 g

Stir Fried Beetroot

Serving: 2

Prep Time: 8 minutes

Cooking Time: 15 minutes

Ingredients

- 2 large sized beetroots
- 2 tablespoon of cold pressed extra virgin olive oil
- 1 teaspoon of Rosemary
- 1 leek stalk, sliced
- 2 tablespoon of fresh, chopped up parsley
- 1 tablespoon of fresh, chopped up chives
- Sea salt as needed
- Pepper as needed

Instructions

Wash up your beetroots and peel them up firs, and then cut them up into halves.

Take a pan and pour in the olive oil and heat it up nicely. Simmer your rosemary and beetroot for 10 minutes with the lid closed up, making sure to keep stirring it from time to time.

Toss in the leeks then and stir them nicely. Pour in about 3 tablespoons of water.

Lock up the lid and cook for yet another 6-8 minutes until the leek is cooked nicely. Toss in the parsley then alongside some chives and keep stirring them finely.

Season them with extra pepper and salt. Serve with some waxy potatoes if you can for added taste.

Nutrition Values

Calories: 166

Fats: 11 g

Carbs: 12 g

Fiber: 5 g

Chapter 7:

Dessert, Snacks and Shakes Recipes

Pumpkin Fries

Serving: 4

Prep Time: 10 minutes

Cooking Time: 30-40 minutes

Ingredients

- 1 piece of pumpkin
- ¼ cup of cold pressed extra virgin olive oil
- 1 teaspoon of sea salt/organic salt
- 1 pinch of curry powder
- 1 pinch of cumin powder

Instructions

Start off by pre-heating your oven to a temperature of 350 degrees Fahrenheit.

Cut up your pumpkins in halves and scoop out the seed and strings inside.

Wash up each individual section of your pumpkin using a sharp knife and peel off the large pieces. Cut up the pulp into fine strips, resembling French fries.

Spread out the pumpkin strips onto a tray and spray them with some olive oil. Season them with some salt, curry powder, pepper and cumin powder.

Bake them for about 30-40 minutes and keep tossing them from time to time.

Serve!

Nutrition Values

Calories: 123

Fats: 4 g

Carbs: 23 g

Fiber: 2 g

Fresh Cherries Mixed With Macadamia Almond Cream

Serving: 2

Prep Time: 12 hours

Cooking Time: 0 minutes

Ingredients

- 10 oz. Macadamia Nuts

- 2 oz. almonds

- 2 cups fresh almond milk

- 1 tablespoon of vanilla powder

- 1 teaspoon of Stevia

- 1 pound of fresh cherries

Instructions

It is best if you use Alkaline Water and soak up your Macadamia nuts alongside the almonds for at least 12 hours.

After 12 hours, take a blender and blend up all of your soaked nuts. Toss in the Stevia, vanilla powder and almond milk, and bring it to a fine paste with a smooth texture.

Toss in just a little bit of almond milk again.

Put it in your fridge and let it sit for about 3 hours and serve the smoothie with some fresh cherries.

Nutrition Values

Calories: 310

Fats: 13 g

Carbs: 13 g

Fiber: 1 g

Indian Vegetable Snack – Aloo Gobi

Serving: 2

Prep Time: 5 minutes

Cooking Time: 10 minutes

Ingredients

- 1 oz. fresh ginger

- 2 cloves of fresh garlic

- 4 green chilies

- 2 large onions

- 14 oz. diced tomatoes

- 2 lbs cauliflower

- 2 teaspoons Turmeric

- 2 teaspoon Garam masala

- 4 oz. cold pressed extra virgin olive oil

- 1/3 cup of coriander and cilantro leaves

- Salt as need

- 1/3 cup of mint

- 2 teaspoon of cayenne pepper

- 3 cups of water

Instructions

Start off by grinding up your garlic, ginger and chili together.

Pour in some oil in a pan and heat it up for 3 minutes.

Toss in the onions and saute them until fully golden.

Add in the paste them and stir them for few seconds.

Toss in the tomatoes, turmeric, salt, Garam Masala, chili and cook until you see that the tomatoes are nicely pulpy with their oil complete separated which should take no more than 5 minutes.

Add in the rest of the ingredients and stir them all for 3 minutes. Add in some water. Cook them until the vegetables are finely done and have a thick sauce.

Serve with some Basmati Rice.

Nutrition Values

Calories: 178

Fats: 5 g

Carbs: 25 g

Fiber: 5 g

The Powerful Hulk Green Shake

Serving: 2

Prep Time: 5 minutes

Cooking Time: 0 minutes

Ingredients

- 1 piece of avocado

- ½ a medium sized cucumber

- 1 cup cabbage

- 1 cup of fresh spinach leaves

- 1 peeled up lime

- 1 tablespoon of Super Greens Powder

- Ice cubes as needed

- Alkaline Water

Instructions

Take all of your ingredients and toss them into your blender. Blend the mixture well.

Pour the whole mixture into a glass and toss in the ice cubes. Pour in enough water to cover the cubes up.

Drink chilled.

Nutrition Values

Calories: 31

Fats: 0g

Carbs: 4g

Fiber: 0g

The Perfect Almond Milk For An Alkaline Diet

Serving: 2

Prep Time: 10 minutes

Cooking Time: 0 minutes

Ingredients

- 4 cups fresh raw almond
- Alkaline Water
- Nylon stocking or any other sieving device

Instructions

Take a bowl and pour in some water.

Toss in the fresh almonds and let them soak overnight.

The next morning, drain those almonds and fill up your blender with about 2 cups of drained almonds.

Add the alkaline water to fill up your blender. The general calculation is that 1/3 of almond will require 2/3 of water. Blend the mixture at maximum speed until the whole mix is finely creamy.

Repeat the process with the remaining almonds, if any.

Take the fine nylon stocking or sieve and pour the prepared milk through it.

Make sure to place a bowl underneath and drain it out completely. Use your finger to force the milk through the string for perfect filtering.

Serve!

Nutrition Values

Calories: 132

Fats: 5g

Carbs: 26g

Fiber: 11g

A Very Lucrative Soy Pudding

Serving: 4

Prep Time: 10 minutes

Cooking Time: 0 minutes

Ingredients

- 1 cup of fresh almond milk (prepared from the previous recipe)

- 2 avocados

- Juice from 1 lime

- 2 scoops of Soy Powder

- 1 package of Stevia

- 6-8 ice cubes

Instructions

Open up the lid of your blender and toss in all of the ingredients into your blender.

Mix them up at full speed until the whole mixture has been turned into a nice and smooth pudding.

Pour in the pudding in a bowl serve chilled.

Nutrition Values

Calories: 324

Fats: 3 g

Chapter 7: Dessert, Snacks and Shakes Recipes

Carbs: 64 g

Fiber: 5 g

A Delicious Mixture of Carrot and Grapefruit

Serving: 1

Prep Time: 10 minutes

Cooking Time: 0 minutes

Ingredients

- 2 carrots

- 1 grapefruit

- 3 oz. Alkaline Water

- 3 Alkaline Water ice cubes

- 2-3 mint leaves

Instructions

Peel up the grapefruit. Depending on the model of your juicer, you are going to need to push it through. Make sure to catch the juice as it is made in a cup.

Wash up your carrots then and trim off the ends.

Push them through the juicer too and collect them in a glass.

Pour both of the juices in a tall sized glass and pour in the water. Mix gently.

Toss in some ice cubes to chill out the mixture.

Decorate with some mint leaves if you want a more lucrative looking shake.

Serve chilled.

Nutrition Values

Calories: 70

Fats: 9 g

Carbs: 16 g

Fiber: 5 g

Fine Pizza Bread for Alkaline Pizza

Serving: 1

Prep Time: 10 minutes

Cooking Time: 0 minutes

Ingredients

- 7 oz of Sunflower seeds
- 3 ½ oz. Flax Seeds
- 2 oz. Sundried tomatoes
- Fresh garlic
- 4 tablespoon cold pressed extra virgin olive oil
- Pinch of salt
- Pinch of pepper
- Alkaline spices of your choice

Instructions

Start off by soaking up your sunflower seeds in a bowl of water for about 4 hours.

Take a mixer and toss in the flax seeds and grind them to a very flour-like powder.

Once the sunflower seeds are soaked up, bring them up and toss them into your mixer as well. Blend these for a few seconds.

Toss in all of the ingredients in a bowl and knead the dough thoroughly using your fingers. Make sure you have a nice consistency, and if you want, then you can always add some olive oil or water.

Create several pizza breads and gently toss them into your dehydrator. Alternatively, if you don't have a dehydrator, then you can always go for an oven.

Keep them there to dehydrate for at least 12 hours.

Now this dough can be used for any future pizza creation of yours using alkaline ingredients.

Nutrition Values

Calories: 251

Fats: 2 g

Carbs: 10 g

Fiber: 0g

The Original Cauliflower Mash

Serving: 2

Prep Time: 15 minutes

Cooking Time: 0 minutes

Ingredients

- 1 whole cauliflower cut up into tiny florets

- 2 cups of Brussels sprouts

- 1 cup of walnuts

- ½ a cup of fresh parsley

- ½ a cup of fresh basil

- 1 clove of garlic

- 1 tablespoon of lemon juice

- 2 tablespoon of olive oil

- ½ teaspoon of bell pepper powder

- Sea salt as needed

- Fresh pepper as needed

Instructions

Start off by placing your previously prepared cauliflower florets in a bowl of saltwater. Leave them until they are finely soft.

In the meantime, you place your Brussels sprouts in another bowl until they are fully firm and ready to be chopped up.

Take another bowl and toss in both of the previous items alongside the walnuts, basil, parsley, garlic, bell pepper powder and mix them well.

Toss the mixture into your blender then and keep blending them until they have a finely mashed potato texture.

Season the mixture with some pepper and salt.

Take a pan and heat up some olive oil alongside some lemon juice. Mix them up.

Gently and evenly place the mash on top of 2 plates and pour the olive oil mixture over the mash.

Serve them up nicely!

Nutrition Values

Calories: 94

Fats: 3 g

Carbs: 15 g

Fiber: 3 g

Chapter 8:

How to Stay Motivated

Most people who decide to start a new way of eating or diet regimen often begin with a lot of psyche about it. They are all pumped up in the beginning as they envision how their bodies and their health are going to be transformed.

Unfortunately, the reality is that the majority of people who make the decision to try out a new diet end up quitting somewhere during the process. In most cases, the reason is a lack of motivation to sustain what they started. Motivation is one of the most important aspects of staying the course with any diet, including the Alkaline Diet. The difference between the person who succeeds in improving their health over time and another who fails lies in the levels of their motivation.

There are times when things will get tough and sticking to the Alkaline Diet will not seem like it is worth it, but these challenging days are exactly those days that you need to keep going. As long as you develop the ability to keep your excitement levels up and refuse to give up, you will achieve your goals.

Chapter 8: How to Stay Motivated

Remember the reasons why you are adopting a clean eating diet in the first place – to lose weight and regain control over your health. Here are 7 ways of staying motivated as you embark on your Alkaline Diet journey:

1. **Just start** – You have to simply resolve that you are going to start eating right today! Stop thinking about how difficult it will be to live with the new diet and just start it. Instead of doing wholesale changes to the way you eat, just start making small changes to the kinds of foods that you consume. You will realize that once you get used to those small steps, making the larger transitions will become easier than you once thought. Nobody who has ever gone on a health-transforming diet ever regretted it afterwards!

2. **Find an accountability partner** – Staying accountable is a great way to make sure that you actually do what you are supposed to do. The first few days are going to be the most difficult, and this transition period is when you will need people around you to hold you accountable. Find friends, family members, social media communities, websites, and forums that will keep you committed throughout. Makes sure that there are people who know you are on the Alkaline Diet and are willing to keep tabs on you to help you stick to it. Nobody wants to look like a failure in front of others, and in this case, this kind of fear is a great motivator.

3. **Practice positive thinking** – Keeping negative thoughts out of our minds is a full-time job. However, it is a battle you must learn to fight every day and win. You must learn to keep track of the kind of thoughts running through your mind. Learn to recognize negative thoughts of how you are never going to lose weight or achieve your goals. Once you have acknowledged these negative thoughts, replace them

with positive ones. Don't try to ignore them as if they don't exist. It won't work. The moment a thought like, "This is just too hard for me," enters your mind, say to yourself, "I can do this. I am going to make it." Positive thinking isn't avoiding the issue, but a way to overcome those toxic mindsets that are likely to derail your process.

4. **Fix your eyes on the prize** – You need to focus on the benefits that you will enjoy once you make the Alkaline Diet a lifestyle. You need to remind yourself of all the benefits of adopting this new living philosophy. The biggest problem most people have when faced with anything that requires them to make a painful change is this - They focus on the sacrifices they have to make rather than the opportunities they have to make a meaningful difference! Will it be difficult to stay the course sometimes? Yes, of course. Remember that the standard Westernized diet contains foods that you have probably grown to love. Parting with some of them will seem like a silly or crazy idea. However, think of the benefits that you will gain rather than how hard things will be. This will keep you energized throughout.

5. **Set goals and use them to keep you excited** – Goal-setting is one secret that helps winners win in the first place. It is very difficult to get to where you are going if you don't create goals for yourself. Why is this important? There is coming a time when you will feel deflated and running low on motivation. At a time such as this, you will have to sit down and start thinking about why you aren't excited anymore. Then you will pull out your list of goals that you made in the beginning, and you will start to read through the things that got you excited in the first place. Ask yourself how you can regain that lost excitement. Why were you passionate about those goals in the beginning?

Use your list of goals to reenergize yourself and light that fire again. The goals belong to you, so do not be afraid to remodel the list a bit if necessary. Make sure that you do it using pen and paper, though. Writing your goals by hand has a way of motivating you more than typing something on a computer.

6. **Find people with similar diet goals** – Unlike the other point about accountability partners, this one is more oriented toward people who are also engaged in similar diets. It is easier to stick to your goals when there is someone else to walk with you through the diet. It could be a friend, relative, spouse, or whatever. You do not even have to be on the same diet or set the same goals. As long as you are both encouraging and pushing each other, you are both going to make it. Go and celebrate every milestone that you achieve together, no matter how small. Just don't cheat on your diet while celebrating!

7. **Have a cheat day, but don't do it two days in a row** – It's human to want to break the rules now and then, especially when it comes to the types of foods to eat. If you happen to skip one day and consume something acidic, then there's no major problem to worry about. The important thing is to reflect on your cheat day and make the resolve to go back to your diet. The Alkaline Diet isn't as stringent as some of the others out there. You get to decide what to eat and in what proportions, just as long as it is alkaline in nature. Remember what we said about maintaining a balance, so some acidic foods once in a while won't kill you. Just know that you shouldn't make it a habit and go back to your former lifestyle.

Staying motivated is all about having the proper mindset. If you can get your mind right, then you will make it in your Alkaline Diet journey.

Conclusion

I really do hope that you enjoyed reading the book as much as I enjoyed writing it. The main aim of this book was to not only introduce you to the world of Alkaline Diet but also give you the opportunity to try out the recipes for yourself and see the changes first hand.

Keep in mind that this is only the tip of the iceberg and there's much more to learn about the Alkaline Diet. Take the time to educate yourself further and begin practicing this dietary philosophy.

Stay blessed and stay healthy!

Resources

www.authoritynutrition.com

www.webmd.com

www.draxe.com

www.alkalinediet.net

www.wikipedia.com

www.globalhealingcenter.com